Dedicated to Reggie Jr. ~Rest in peace little one Rest in Peace. Mommy and Daddy Love You.

Table of Contents:

Thanks

Introduction

Lesson #1: You Can Have Your Dream Job

Lesson #2: Getting the Job and Career Advancement: Sometimes It's More About Who You Know, Rather Than What You Know

Lesson #3: General Nursing Knowledge Can Practically be Used Outside the Acute Care Setting

Lesson #4: Nursing Chooses You, You Don't Choose It

Lesson #5: Foundations of the Profession: Integrity, Honesty, Trust, and Creating a Lasting Legacy

Lesson #6: Delegation- Making Sure It's Done Right, Not Again

Lesson #7: Know Your Worth (Branding)

Lesson #8: Know Your Brand, Protect Yourself; Losing Your Nursing License is Not an Option

Lesson #9: Affirmation Comes From Home (The power of a good support network)

Lesson #10: Frequently Asked Questions

Bonus: Crisis Prevention/Intervention Plan

Scriptures to Inspire

References

About

Thanks

Without my husband Reggie Ward after Christ of course, you would not be reading this book. He believed in me when I didn't believe in myself, encouraged me, guided me, and helped me not be so crazy throughout this process. Compartmentalizing-he taught me is the key. Thank you for your unwavering support, love, and never giving up. I hope to make you proud to be my hubby for a very long time. I love you Papi.

Then there is Jocelyn "DJ" McKenzie who encouraged me to start a blog, believed in me, and helped me edit like crazy. I love you girl.

To my mom, my sister Alyssa and my dad, Thank You. Each of you made me who I am. To Mother W and Annette thank you both for all your prayers and encouragement.

To my nursing buddies - we have been through a lot Thank You for believing, encouraging, and contributing to this book in your unique and special ways.

To the nurses I've met online and along the way Thank You.

To Dr. Kim, Thank You for allowing me to quote your work, your kind words and prompt responses to my inquiry.

To my friends and family Thank You. Your support and love means so much to me. I could not have done it without you.

And to you who are reading this page Thank You. I wrote this for you. I was once in your shoes and in a lot of ways still am, at the precipice ready to embark on a new journey- unsure where I will land.

To my church family Christ Fellowship Tampa Thank You, especially to our leadership Bruce and Heather Moore. Always believing, praying, encouraging, and pushing me to do more. You are awesome people.

And last but certainly not least to Jesus who came to earth, lived a sinless life among men, died on the cross for all our sins, and rose again. Thank You! I cannot even begin to describe the love, compassion, and grace you have shown me on my journey. There have been many times I wanted to stop but you birthed this idea in me and are blessing it to succeed. Amen.

Introduction

Welcome! In these pages, you will find lessons my friends and I learned outside the classroom. There are ten lessons that consistently repeated themselves throughout the beginning of my nursing journey. Some of them I wish I had learned before nursing school; nonetheless I'm glad I learned them anyway. These are not the only lessons you will learn. In fact, I'm still learning from these and other lessons today. I graduated from Nursing school unemployed, (by choice) bored, depressed, and seriously considering working in a hospital even though I love public health nursing and desired to work elsewhere.

However, God blessed me with a great job and I initially started writing mostly to heal during that first crazy and emotionally challenging year. From that and other experiences came this book. Read what speaks to you, in any order you choose. I hope you enjoy my take on things through a Christ centered lens.

Lesson #1: **You Can Have Your Dream Job**

You know when you're in nursing school and in class learning about patient care or you're in psychology learning how benzodiazepines decrease anxiety or in medical surgical nursing learning the importance of the kidneys only after you just failed or barely pass the exam.... It is in that moment that you question your purpose for being here…in nursing school and if there is a type of nursing area that you will be able to excel in? Well I am here to tell you, YES! There is a nursing specialty for each and every one of us no matter how diverse we can be.

A few Types of Nursing:

- Ambulatory
- Cardiac
- Critical Care
- Nurse Manager
- Public Health
- Community Health
- Informatics
- Writer/ Entrepreneur
- Consultant

- Educator
- Professor
- Psychiatric
- Rehabilitative
- Telephonic
- Advocate (Explore Specialties,9/19/2013)

And the list goes on… you are only limited by your imagination!!! These and more nursing specialties can be found here: https://www.discovernursing.com/explore-specialties#no-filters

The Bottom Line: If you are meant to be a nurse, then there is a field where you will shine and be able to make a difference in someone's life. The beauty of nursing is that if you are living your passion and I am living mine, we come together holistically helping the client. At the end of the day this is why we joined this profession, to help people! Sometimes you find your niche outside the classroom. That's where I found mine.

Lesson #2: Getting the Job and Career Advancement: Sometimes It's More About Who You Know, Rather Than What You Know

It really is a matter of perspective. Before I delve into how I got started as a public health nurse leading me to become a nurse writer let me start with a few comments, statements and "encouragement"... (*And I use this term loosely*) that I've received along the way:

- **"You have to work in the hospital for two years and get experience."**- This makes sense if I was planning to work in the hospital but I was not.
- **"Once you get your two years at the bedside, then you probably want to work in labor and delivery in the hospital and/or pediatrics and then apply to a public health nursing job."**

Why would I want to do that? Let's think about this. My plan is to be a public health nurse in every sense of the word working with the public in their communities and helping them to prevent acute care events as much as possible. So, this statement makes me think of going to heck and back to pursue my God given passion. By engaging in an activity I loathe(I know it's a strong word) I increase my chances of **A)** Not making it out of the hospital unscathed- likely burnt-out and **B)** wasting precious time when I could actually be pursuing my dreams!!!

- **"Are you a nurse/ what do you do?"** I have heard this statement many times when I explain/ it's known:

    A) I do not work in a hospital and

    B) My passion is preventative medicine which means I do not start Ivs and pass meds all day which in the right settings is necessary just not in my field.

- **"Why don't work in the hospital? There is *"good money"* in the hospital."** This may be true but in my opinion and for me the increased stress and pressure would be more than any compensation I could make. My philosophy has always been if you follow your passion THE MONEY WILL COME.

If You or I listen to these comments and other people, professors', colleagues', and families' personal opinions regarding our nursing career we may never have a nurse working in an ambulatory care center or in their communities.

So enough about "encouraging words" here's a little background of my nursing journey:

I was sitting in my community health class and it just clicked….made "my heart smile" like a dear person I know says. I have always wanted to help people, prevent disease, increase wellness, and to encourage people to utilize the hospital in acute settings, hence community health nursing is a perfect fit for me. The challenge was landing a public health job. A few of years ago when I was in nursing school the system was set up that I would work in the hospital for two years and then I was "free" to pursue my dreams in nursing. The problem with this logic is that while working for two years in something I may not be remotely interested in I would miss the opportunity to gain experience in a field of personal interest and meaning.

So, I chose to turn down a nursing internship starting off nice at the area's level one trauma/teaching hospital and pursue other avenues. Now it took some work. I had to plan ahead and follow the desire God had given me. One day, I took my roommate at the time to community health training. I felt very down about not having a job yet and all around crummy since most of my graduating class had already been working for several months. At this training, "Nurse J", a nurse from the local health department was presenting and describing her job. God placed on my heart that I speak to her after the meeting. I reluctantly shared with her my passion for public health nursing after she informed me of her start in the field. "Nurse J" must have sensed my love for this specialty because she said something along the lines of "We need a young passionate nurse like you in the field.... You would have to pass the state boards first and then apply for a job at a local health department but you might not get it due to experience." I shadowed "Nurse J" and called her from time to time. Well, it just so happens (only God), I passed my NCLEX exam right around the time available positions at the counties' clinics were posted. I applied to two positions. Lo and Behold---since, I had been talking to "Nurse J", she told the supervisor that I applied and my passion for Public Health Nursing.

Throughout this process, "Nurse J" reiterated that she could not get me a job. Eventually, I received a phone interview, followed by a face –to- face and tour (when offered a tour after an interview, always a good sign:)) for one of the clinics. I became the youngest Senior Registered Nurse with the County's Health Department serving as the Women's Team Lead and a new graduate at that. Exactly four months after graduation, I landed my dream job!!! If I had not spoken to that nurse and cultivated that mentor relationship or listened more closely to my "encouragers" I would not be writing today (more about networking in the Lesson # 10).And even though years have passed and things have changed I am forever grateful for those who gave me a chance and for that position which has catapulted me to where I am today.

As a profession, nursing is about connecting with people so it makes sense to use this same principle when looking for employment or advancement. Advancement comes in many forms: monetary, responsibility, authority, or sometimes an increase and combination of all these things. For example: While I was working at my assigned clinic, clinic A, an opening became available at the County's busiest clinic, Clinic B. A few weeks later, I was called into the clinic's administrator's office and offered the position. It was a lateral promotion that allowed me to lead a busier Women's Health Clinic. Although, I did not know it at the time, God is crafty that way. He set it up so the steady pace I was working at in Clinic A prepared me for the workflow at Clinic B. It came with some challenges but it increased my skills and was a great opportunity. I also enjoyed working for my new supervisor. These positions opened my eyes to a subspecialty I hadn't considered before; Women's' Health, all I knew when I signed up was I needed to follow my dreams.

The Bottom Line: Relationships are key in this profession. Without them, I would not have landed my dream job, been promoted, or able to expand my influence as a public health nurse today. Just remember, judge for yourself the character of a person and cultivate those relationships you deem worthy, as we all have different experiences that we can learn from. (See more in FAQ Lesson).

Lesson #3: General Nursing Knowledge Can Practically be Used Outside the Acute Care Setting

When we graduate, we are generalists. We are taught an overview on a myriad of nursing topics so that when we enter the workforce we will be malleable in whatever setting we're in. Now, if your school is like most, in addition to a general overview there is a tilt toward acute care nursing for the first two years after graduation. With that said, personally I was scared because of that tilt that when branching out I would not be able to do any other type of nursing; Unless of course, I followed the prescription and got my two years of bedside nursing, then maybe I could do it. I soon learned just like any career even when you start as a generalist, you get hands-on/ on-the-job training that you can assimilate into your fundamental nursing skills.

Do not believe the hype- that you must understand every concept now or you won't be a good nurse. Whether you're going to work in the ER, ICU, acute care, correctional facility, or school health, there will be training and time to specialize after graduation. Just make sure it is the training you deserve and is extensive enough to meet your needs. So, while in school do not over work yourself if you do not remember every color description of drainage from Jackson-Pratt® drain because:

1) Things have a funny way of coming to you when you need them,

2) If this is a part of a regular assessment you will be doing, you will have lots a practice and experience and

3) There will be/make time to ask lots of questions before it is show time.

Enjoy learning nursing concepts overall. In the long run, this will help you set a great generalist foundation to work from. If you don't believe me, believe this: I went from working at a Women's Health Clinic to a Substance Abuse /Mental Health Residential Facility to Home Visiting in Public Health - all with a generalist's degree.

The Bottom Line: Strong Foundation equals Strong Nurses.

Lesson #4: Nursing Chooses You, You Don't Choose It

Now the title of this lesson might sound crazy because yes, of course we are able to choose our own destiny. But is that statement really true? Can we choose burgers over fries, a smoothie over a salad, mustard over mayo? Why, yes of course! The point is if you're actively choosing nursing for reasons such as money, fame, or prestige, then you will soon find yourself very bitter. Through personal experiences and those of others in this profession I have learned not having a passion for helping people at your core will very quickly become problematic. We see how motive affects career in the lives of two nursing students Selma and Victoria.

Selma and Victoria both want to be nurses. Selma is intrigued about having the option of always being employable (this as we will or have already learned is not necessarily true) and making between $50,000- $70,000 at an entry level position. Victoria on the other hand comes to nursing because of something that happened at church one day. She was in the pew when one of the parishioners grabbed their chest, at first no one noticed and although Victoria did she was very scared. Immediately, her brain flipped to helping the person with the skills she learned at a recent CPR training. She was able to get the member emergency help and forever ignite her passion to help people in acute situations.

I can relate to Victoria .Originally, I wanted to be an Obstetrician/Gynecologist. I just thought being a doctor was very prestigious and I wanted to deliver babies. This dream changed when my grandfather who lived across the country passed away. Usually, no matter how many years have passed, fifteen to be exact, I cannot tell how I came to nursing without crying. More about that later.

Both Selma and Victoria attend the same nursing school but have vastly different experiences. Where Victoria excels and/or copes with setbacks by drawing on her passion for caring for clients in imminent situations; Selma continues to forcefully propel herself through with the promise of fame, riches, and recognition. Selma becomes irritable and stressed, so much so she's cutting corners in her studies, while Victoria's' confidence and competence is increasing in addition to her feelings of joy, peace, and satisfaction knowing. She knows she is right where she's supposed to be. Eventually, Selma graduates but it was a treacherous road. She lands an entry level position but resigns after six months due to depression and overall burned out feeling. Victoria lands an entry level position in the ER internship program and loves it.

Both have bad days but what they were able to draw upon in those bad days is what did or did not get them through. When we decide not to follow our passion, we set ourselves up to fail. We waste time, energy, resources, and overall hutzpah to get the job done. Follow your own star, stay in your lane, ask God to order your steps these statements/ sayings mean the same thing, do whatever it is that brings you joy. Whether it be nursing, psychology, entrepreneurship, nutrition, or working in the entertainment field. Anything that makes our heart sing is what we should be doing. The money, fame, and recognition will come but the peace of mind, joy, and calm that come from following your journey is invaluable. If you do not think so, remember this: your passion will keep appearing until you pursue it. It is up to you when you take the plunge and start the real work of making it a daily, hourly, minute by minute reality.

I personally, have been Selma and Victoria at different points in my nursing career. I have seen and experienced too many Selma's; taking out their lack of passion on clients in their most vulnerable state: navigating the healthcare system. At some points, I pursued what others have told me or what I felt would be a good fit , although it is ok to try things out and learn something new, once you see it is not working , pray and if led, go on to what He has called you too. God has a life far beyond your dreams planned for you. (Jeremiah 29:11 NKJV)

My passion for nursing came from family tragedy. My grandfather lived on the west coast and I on the east, so I saw him every few years. He became ill and needed a heart transplant which he received and was doing well. He even stopped smoking. Eventually, his body started to reject the organ and in the middle of the night one evening my mom received that dreaded call: the one where she learned her father had gone on to glory. When I heard my mother break down, it triggered an emotion in me. You never know how much someone meant until they are gone. The only solace I have till this day is remembering when I talked to my grandpa before he passed how highly he spoke of the nurses that were treating him, like he was their family. In that tragic moment, I knew although I was unable to say goodbye and although I never met those angels; I knew that my grandfather received the best care and love possible. From that moment on, I wanted to be a nurse.

When I was rejected from my alma mater once, told to pick another major and then attend the accelerated program, placed number seven on the waitlist the second time, disrespected and manipulated by professors, harassed, threatened to not graduate, bullied by coworkers, burnout, given a second chance, moved on, and given another great opportunity, I held on to my core passion of wanting to treat those I serve like family just as my grandfather was treated.

The Bottom Line: Without passion as your core to enter and sustain in this profession: it will be hard to succeed much less enjoy nursing.

Lesson #5: Foundations of a Profession: Integrity, Honesty, Trust, and Creating a Lasting Legacy

Nursing is not a job; it is a profession and if you consider it more of the former than latter please reread Lesson # 4 or go directly to Lesson # 10. If you consider what a profession is versus a job you will note two very distinct paths. A job is something you do on a regular basis just like a career except when you resign, quit, or are terminated that's it. You move on to the next thing. In a career these things will happen but the passion for the industry never leaves you. So your profession is worth protecting.

The four principles of creating an unshakeable foundation for your nursing career are integrity, honesty, trust, and a lasting legacy. These principles must be ever present in your mind and spirit in every nursing action you do. Now does this mean before you give an injection you will think to yourself integrity…honesty and so on? No! It does mean you will embody these characteristics in every nursing action you do.

Integrity:

According to the Merriam Webster Dictionary Online: Dictionary and Thesaurus (9/23/13) integrity is "firm adherence to a code of especially moral or artistic values: Incorruptibility". This means doing what is right even if it is not popular. If you or someone made an error and you immediately stop and correct the action so that the client's safety is intact, that's integrity. You may think no one will know but **you** will know. Once you have compromised, it is hard to recover. I know this very well.

I had a preceptor in the ICU who was about to pass medication and a package of medicine dropped on the floor. In that moment she naturally picked them up and discarded them and redrew more from the Pixis®. Who wants meds off a hospital floor?!!? She documented why she was getting more medication and then we continued on. This taught me two very valuable lessons. First, the public has rightly so ranked nursing as one if not the most trusted profession in the USA. Secondly, I learned integrity is natural. The nurse did not make a big show of what happened. She just did what she knew to be right which taught me, an impressionable nursing student, that this was someone to model my behavior after as someone who truly embodies integrity.

Honesty:

Sometimes, the truth is not welcomed but very much warranted. You know who you are as a nurse and a person. If you do not make this known to others who have influence over / around your career, then you will end up being an unhappy nurse not doing what you love. At the same token, clients may not want to hear they need to take care of themselves but, they will respect that you care enough to tell them the truth regarding their situation. Countless times I have seen clients go unassisted medically because the professional does not broach the subject. I do not pretend to have all the answers or know what to say in every situation but we all took an oath and part of the oath is to help people heal. How then can we help them if we do not broach the tough/ awkward subjects such as feminine odor, morbid obesity, or mental health needs?

I have been the professional and the client and basically it isn't easy telling someone things need to change for better health but it must be done. Imagine how many less tragedies, medical setbacks, and errors could be avoided with open communication between clients and providers. I strongly believe communication is the key. I would rather have a client mad because I privately approached them about a symptom I noted and suggested be further investigated by a higher level medical professional than to find out I just let the client go, the symptom progresses to a pelvic inflammatory disease because a STI was never treated and now the client has the possibility of high-risk pregnancies.

I have sat across from the doctor and had he/she tell me to lose weight, my symptoms are stress related, and/or I have anxiety and I hated every minute of it. No one, especially someone in the field; wants to be told they are not "normal" but after reflection I respected their honesty/ professional opinion and have also had clients thank me because I cared enough to tell them when, why, and how to get help. Honesty is always best and strengthens the bond between client and provider no matter what is happening.

Trust:

Trust according to the Merriam Webster Dictionary Online: Dictionary and Thesaurus (9/23/13) is "[…] reliance on the character, ability, strength, or truth of someone or something." If you don't believe in yourself, how can you expect others too?

In nursing school, they use to tell us to "fake it till you make it." Now one might wonder how this can practically be done. In essence, this means submerging yourself in your career and actively learning all you can even nuances, so then one day you look back and are able to teach /show the ropes to someone else. A couple of ways I suggest submerging yourself that I found helpful include:

- ✓ not taking any or minimal days off the first ninety days of the job,
- ✓ ask lots of questions until you understand,
- ✓ volunteer for new projects or committees, and
- ✓ remember this is practice and practice makes perfect.

These foundational skills will help build your confidence and competence making you a readily trusted authority in your choice nursing field. That's what it's all about. Your confidence will enable you to succeed in getting the job done successfully.

Legacy:

In Mathew 6:16 Jesus says" You will know them by their fruits." If that is the case, it stands to reason in your nursing career what impacts you've made; your legacy is your fruit. I for one want a legacy rich with character, perseverance, and adventure for those who follow in my steps. That means being diligent in my work, having integrity, honesty, and trust. What type of legacy would you like to leave?

When someone mentions your name or you ask for a recommendation you want them not to lack positive attributes to describe you. The only way this can and will happen is being honest with yourself first and then truly embracing your role in nursing, having the courage to face all challenges head-on no matter what the outcome, and trusting the training and experiences that you have had in and since nursing school. This open letter from a nurse to her community sums legacy up:

A Nurses Legacy By: Raqui Ward 5/9/2013

"Dear Community,

I leave you today for greener meadows, for a triumphant return to peace for my body is weary and my mind is filled with many memories. Some good, bad... indifferent but nonetheless memories.

Although I leave, be of good cheer as I am not gone, just absent in body. My spirit of care lives on...

You see that little girl running around enjoying her adoptive family...or the young mother breastfeeding her baby? What about the nurse practitioner you saw today...that took the time to get to know you? She was in a class I taught about compassion.

Aunt Jane understands that she takes the yellow pills twice a day and the green one at night because I took the extra time to make sure she had her medication right.

Maybe you met the nurse anesthetist that prepped you before surgery - I befriended her, telling her the sky was the limit despite her current circumstances and she dared to believe it.

The nurse day in and day out helping you in rehab? Well, he and I connected online through blogging and now the rehab app he created keeps all your progress in one place, at the fingertips of you and your family.

Did you meet your child's teacher? I told her that being a teenage mother was just the beginning of her story. I inspired her to go to school and provide for her family.

So you see, I'm still here in my words, actions, deeds, and planted seeds. My spirit of care lives on and now it's up to you to carry the legacy of care on.

Thank you for allowing me the opportunity to care for, inspire, and encourage you. It was my pleasure and now I rest; knowing the legacy I leave serves as a catalyst to the next generation of caring.

Take Care,

~Raqui"

I pray this inspires you.

The Bottom Line: If your nursing profession is not built on a solid foundation everything you worked for is in jeopardy.

Lesson #6: Delegation- Making Sure It's Done Right, Not Again

There is a saying I picked up …you guessed it… outside of nursing school at one of my clinical experiences. A wise nurse once said something to the effect, "On this floor, our motto is if you don't do it right [the first time] when will you have time to do it over again?"

This is powerful. Go back and read that again. This lesson literally gave my nursing career a paradigm shift. Before this I was so busy focusing on getting the task done and checking it off my list. But, he was right; just because it is checked off my list does not make it right.

That is how it is when it comes to delegation. I have been there when you are burnt-out to a little crisp and it is all you can do as a nurse to let your support staff to do something you would be better suited to do although within their scope of practice. It is in those moments you must consider with whom and with what you are placing your clients' wellbeing in. If you wouldn't trust that person to water a plant-you certainly can't trust them to pass meds?!!!!! On the flip side, you need help. I do not care how many classes and books and experience you have, we are not islands to ourselves. We all need help and you are going to have to trust somebody. Yes, you can complete all the items on your list, but not successfully.

So how do you know who, what, when, and where to delegate? Well it's very scientific… you see, it's called the gut test. Within a few minutes of meeting someone you can pretty much sum them up. Now that does not mean you know them like you know the mole on your left shoulder but you have a pretty good judge of their character. In my opinion with practice and time, you will get better and better. It took me a long while to become comfortable with certain "habits" staff had with clients but after some self-reflection and a few kick in the pants of caring the load solo, I understood that we all have our way of doing things and I have to be okay as long as the same quality results for the client. You will know as a nurse who can do what and how effectively by trusting your nursing instinct. It is there, some call it intuition; regardless, trust your gut. I'll say it again; **TRUST YOUR GUT** or you'll be the one doing it again.

Delegation Tips:

- ✓ Genuinely get to know staff on a personal and professional level
- ✓ Be cool
- ✓ Relax
- ✓ Start delegating small task within the persons scope of practice building to larger tasks within that same scope as time progresses
- ✓ Be **direct** and **specific** about the help you need

- ✓ Nurse to Nurse delegation needs to be handled professionally
- ✓ Speak to your coworker/ colleagues how you would like to be spoken to.
- ✓ The hospitality / housekeeping staff are a part of your team genuinely get to know them and work with them as well(in any setting)
- ✓ Remember it may not be done exactly how you would have done it but what matters is quality

The Bottom Line: Either do it right/ delegate it right the first time or plan to do it again... usually when your already swamped with no way to win.

Lesson #7: Know Your Worth (Branding)

This by far is the toughest lesson I had to learn. They say things of emotional significance are highly memorable and with this lesson it is true. Hopefully, the pain I went through will help you avoid this major pitfall.

When we devalue ourselves, we set ourselves up for a lot of sleepless nights, anxiety, and heartache. I love public health nursing, no matter what the stats, outlook, joys, or triumphs there is no other niche in nursing I'd rather be. With that said, I also live in a reality in which I need to provide for my family, pay my bills, and hopefully leave the world better than when I entered it. Sometimes, the passion for the niche out shadows the reality of our self-worth and sometimes others have to remind us of this. I had to learn that I am valuable; I am an excellent nurse, sharp, quick study, and good at what I do. What are some adjectives that best describe you?

It is not cocky or conceited to value yourself, your skills, or what you have to bring to the table. Too often society wants everyone to be the same and no one pushes or shoves in "line" because it is not polite and it will hurt somebody's feelings. Well, I'm here to tell you it is not a crime. People are like a business; you must market, maintain, and enhance your business. Nurses, we are the business. What have you done for your business (yourself) in one of the categories of building, maintaining, or enhancing lately? If you're not doing anything, then you just exist and what kind of existence is that?

In nursing countless people fill our heads that we will:

1) always have a job and
2) make "good money"…

These statements are true some of the time for some of the people. I have been on both ends of the spectrum making squat to making a comfortable living. But, it was not until I recognized that I was not valuing myself, or my business correctly that it really stung, Nursing didn't recognize me. Hello! **Wake-up Call**. Nobody is going to recognize someone just existing .Nursing is a great profession for those who are compassionate, passionate, analytical, and enthusiastic but making $17/hour going on three years of experience is not going to cut it.

At this point I'm sure you are thinking to yourself "That will never happen to me." How many times have we as nurses heard patients say the same thing? Well, I too thought and believed people; especially fellow nurses, would be honest and look out for my best interest. How naïve! There are those out there that help the next generation but the majority is looking out for their interest because hey, they have to eat too. The key problem with my theory was expecting someone else to look out for me. This only happens when you're a baby, in a good relationship/marriage, or friendship. Other than that, outside your family, proceed with caution!

Look out for yourself by remembering the adjectives you used to describe yourself earlier.

Steps to knowing your worth and getting paid for it:

1. Take inventory of your experiences from nursing or elsewhere; including leadership, training, volunteerism, and advocacy. This could be your resume.
2. Type up a commercial or snap shot of the attributes that makes you an awesome nurse. You are awesome! Do not limit yourself to quote unquote "nursing skills"
3. Recite/memorize these attributes so that when necessary you can portray them
4. Recognize your value to an organization/group/field and tweak that information to fit your snapshot to enhance your negotiation skills
5. Research, Research, Research…a simple online search about your filed of interest, the current benefits, ins and outs, salary and talking to those in the industry or specific field are valuable. Know your goals, plans,

and lifestyle needs and consider these when looking to make a career change and in the negotiation phase.

6. Compile all above data and internalize so you are prepared for negotiations.

7. Do not negotiate until an offer is made. Watch out for interviewers who offer pigeon hole offers or evade negotiation saying "there is no room for negotiation" or "this is the offer" both are not true there is always room to negotiate you may not get everything or anything you want but speak your peace. Use lines such as "you are our best candidate" to your advantage. For instance saying "As the best candidate I would expect/accept..."

8. Once an offer is made **a)** say thank you but you need time to think about it **b)** Negotiate offer with the previous information you complied in steps 5 and 6. Be direct about your needs increase salary, flexibility, time, and other needs **c)** Know what your bottom line is (use previous offers as a reference point) What is the minimum you are willing to accept. Max? Mid-range? Be willing to compromise reasonably stating, "I would expect ...based on...." While still being direct and to the point.

9. Accept offer on your terms, theirs, or walk away.

10. Be confident in your decision

11. Practice makes perfect- you may not always get what you want but you will the next time.

12. Walk through all pros and cons of job and use this information in negotiations

13. **Get it in writing!!!!!**

14. Pray for peace about the decision.

The Bottom Line: You are a business. Know your worth and don't let anybody take it away from you.

Lesson #8: Know Your Brand, Protect Yourself; Losing Your Nursing License is Not an Option!

As this lesson suggest losing your nursing license is not a joke. I use to be very cavalier on this topic but once I wised up and really let that sink in I came to one conclusion. Protect my license at all cost. How do you do that? By taking care of yourself.

I have always lived and work by the philosophy that in order to care for others I must take care of myself. Now, there are people who will try to make you feel bad for this or even selfish but it's not. **Let me repeat.** It is not selfish to care for yourself or use self-preservation. In fact, it is selfish for you not to do so. Why you ask? Because without you, there is no one to investigate nursing homes, care for the sick, pass medications, notice a subtle change in a client that could mean the difference between life or death to the untrained or weary eyes, no one to sing to the ICU patient, or talk her daughter through a DNR. When you are "off", it throws everybody off; so take care of yourself nurse, Take Care. <ins>**In fact, if you only read this chapter, your patients, co-workers, clients, family, friends, and you will thank you.**</ins>

Now that I have completely berated you, let's talk about the practicality of this. In the fast pace, instant gratification world no one wants to hear "I need a bathroom break", "I haven't had lunch", or "I'm sick" but the fact of the matter is *(although I do not have scientific evidence to back this up save my own experiences and that of others)* nurses who take care of themselves are more productive. How can you pass medications or insert that Foley properly if all you can think about is how full your bladder is and your stomach is running on empty. Also ask yourself why it is such a big trend to talk about taking care of **You** in medicine?

Have we lost it? Since when did not taking care of you become a novel idea? Again, a simple internet search will lend a myriad of results related to self-preservation, burnout prevention, and nurse coaching. Let's get back to basics!

I have come up with a plan I personally use to take care of myself so that I may take care of others and have also written about under my pin name Raqui Ward on my blog http://horizions.blogspot.com/ multiple times. Below are some new and expounded upon concepts for Take Care Nursing.

Take-Care Nurse Tips:

1. **Arrive early rather than leave late**- This is a very important concept and may not be conducive in all settings. Usually, if you get an early start on the day you can wrap up things early or on time.

2. **Keep the golden hour clear as much as possible for emergencies** - It never fails that the first hour of the day and last hour are always crazy. It is when your post-op patient returns after being gone all day, a mother of a chronic asthmatic child walks into the clinic for the" five o'clock triage", a man that has been coughing up a lung for the better part of a week decides to brighten your door, or the post-partum mom calls about a fever she has had for three days. Now I'm sure your experiences have been with more or less extreme cases. I must admit some circumstances are unavoidable. The golden hours of morning, lunch, and end of shift is when stuff happens. So prepare your day ahead as much as possible for these emergencies, admissions, discharges, and other things that pop up. It may not work in every case but, my experiences have been most of the time it will.

3. **Cut the balloon-** In nursing school, I was a very stressed out little person, especially at my nursing internship so I sought professional counseling. If it takes a professional to make it through, I highly recommend it. It is comforting to have an unbiased person to talk to and see how silly some of the things we think about ourselves are out loud. I say all this because in these sessions, I learned the concept of cutting the balloon. Now I must admit, I did not fully get

or incorporate this concept until I got out of nursing school. Even after several attempts, I have to change my routine every now and then. Cutting the balloon means once you clock out, walk off that floor or remove your badge, it is finished. Whatever happened or didn't is done. Yes, it's hard. Again, I am a work in process on this one. I will say once I intentionally started doing this, I was so much happier and able to be a more effective nurse and functioning human being. Ways I cut the balloon or to wind down include:

- ✓ not answering emails etc. the last 15 or so minutes of my day,
- ✓ listening to my favorite cd or audio book on the drive to and from work,
- ✓ driving home a different way,
- ✓ going to the gym after work, and
- ✓ doing something with my hands once I get home that I don't normally do while working, such as latch hooking or painting. It works, and the benefits are endless. How do you wind down after a hard day's work?

4. **Embrace non-nursing friends-** It is a real blessing to talk to someone who is not in the field because you don't end up just talking about nursing. Also, if you are like me and have some really awesome nursing friends, try intentionally to connect with them on a different

level. For instance I have one friend that I walk with, another who likes to dance, and another I can talk about spirituality with. The key is balance, of course when you put nurses together we are going to talk about nursing , don't try to fight it, embrace it but also talk about other things such as hobbies or interest.

5. **Balance-**This goes without saying but balanced nutrition, exercise, sleep, and stress management are key.

6. **Under promise and over deliver-**I'm sure you've heard this before, I know I have. When you over promise and under deliver you create a reputation you might not be ready to defend. This way if you end up doing more than was required you get looked at as going above and beyond. You know yourself, your time management, and your limits! Be honest with yourself and your coworkers. You will be surprised how people like the truth.

7. **Be proactive-** You are the CEO of your health and well-being. No one will take care of you as well as you do.

For more tips check out the Take Care posts on my blog.

The Bottom Line: You cannot help anyone if you have not first taken care of you. Your efforts may be well intentioned, pious even, but eventually your body, mind, spirit, and those around you will say enough is enough! Take care of yourself!

Lesson #9: Affirmation Comes From Home (The power of a good support network)

In 2012 I attended the "Women Heal Thyself: Mind. Body, Spirit conference hosted by the Florida Minority Health Promotion Network Inc. at the University of South Florida in which Dr. Kimberly Ventus-Darks from drkimspeaks.com said something that revolutionized my life. "Our place of employment is not a place for personal therapy or understanding. When they hired you they expected you to already be complete." She went on to say affirmation comes from home.

This literally changed my life. Too often I look for approval of God's plan for me as a nurse at the workplace. You may be thinking what is wrong with that? Doesn't that make sense, since you are a nurse? That's what I thought, but the problem with this thinking is that when you are praised at work you become really happy and when you are corrected, you become very sad or upset and bring that home with you. Think about the earlier quote by Dr. Kim saying. **"[Your] place of employment is not a place for personal therapy...they expected you to already be complete."** Meaning whatever issues you have such as abandonment, anger management, self-esteem, anxiety, fear, hyperactivity will not get solved on a 12 hour, 9am-5pm, or even overnight shift.

Sure, you may make "friends" but lasting relationships are built when you are being yourself and not someone you are supposed to be. When you come home to a supportive environment, the waxing and waning days of work will not affect you because your confidence is rooted in truth; the truth you learned at home through your support network. It is important to surround yourself with other nurses and non-nurses, your family, your faith, your friends, and whomever or whatever else you believe positively impacts you. This creates balance and a balanced person is a more effective nurse... and in my experience the correction days will decrease if you focus on your support network. This concept is the complete opposite of nursing school when I attended, in that we were taught to eat, breath, and bathe nursing.

In fact, I remember nursing orientation like it was yesterday. On that day, they told us to say goodbye to our lives essentially for the next two years of school because we could not and would not have lives, and to say goodbye to our loved ones and family. How ridiculous!!!!!!!!!! Yes, nursing is a serious trusted profession and no matter where we work, we hold lives in the balance. And yes, you must be a focused, driven-, and a purposed person to succeed in this field. But what of this success, if after the end of obtaining it, you have nothing to show for it, nor anyone to share it with. I am glad I was placed in my cohort; there were many married, engaged, and/ or with kids during this time and they managed to succeed. I'm sure if you ask them it was not easy. Heck, I was neither a wife, fiancée, nor a mother while being a student and it was tough on me. Even people who prefer to keep to themselves have at least one person they confide in; we all succeeded with the important people in our lives.

The Bottom Line: Life is a Merry Go round not a teeter-totter ☺

Lesson #10: Frequently Asked Questions

1. What if I found out nursing is not for me?

Hopefully, you have taken the time to do some real soul searching as to why you want to be a nurse. If you come to the conclusion that it is because of the money, easy to find job, stable & growing job market, then you might want to keep searching .While the above is true some of the time, It is not true all the time and for everybody. Speaking from personal experience, when I was unemployed once I had someone state" I've never known a nurse who couldn't find a job". This is where having passion for the field carries you through. Refer back to Lesson # 4.

2. How do I balance self, family, friends, and school obligations? I feel like I always need to study!!!!!!

Studying is important but studying to the point of exhaustion is unwise. There are only so many hours in a day and if you do not take out time for self-care, care of others, and relationships in your life, it will catch up with you. Refer back to Lesson #8.

I would also be remiss if I did not mention the NCLEX examination in this conversation. Yes. This is an important test, one in which your future will be determined as far as your nursing license. With that said, once you have prepared be done. There is such a thing as over preparing to the point of mental and/or physical exhaustion. My advice is to at minimum least the day before the test is do activities you enjoy rather than studying up unto the last minute not giving your brain a chance to rest.

3. **How do I maintain my nursing network?**

Throughout your nursing career you will meet fellow students, faculty, staff, nurses, and others in the nursing industry that will be beneficial to your future success. First you must determine who is for you. To do this you must ask yourself three questions:

1) *Do I like, enjoy, and/or admire this person and why?* This question is the basis for a successful networking relationship. It is easier to maintain contact with someone you have something in common with rather than forcing a relationship with someone you do not.

2) *How will my association with them add to my nursing repertoire and vice versa*? A successful relationship depends on symbiosis or mutual respect in which both parties have some of their needs met.

3) *How much effort will be needed to maintain this relationship*? There is no right answer except that you must weigh the cost and benefits of maintaining this relationship and consider if you are ready and able to put in the amount of effort it requires.

Once you answer these questions and the person meets your basic criteria then it's simply a matter of building a foundation from what you already have in common with them. A genuine foundation and relationship is more successful. The person will mutually be interested in you if you meet their criteria as well and things will naturally blossom on their own.

The first question is especially essential; because if you genuinely enjoy how, what, who, and where the person is going, then connecting will not be a chore. I suggest at minimum, following up with the person once a quarter, filling them in on your life and asking about theirs. When you need something is not the time to say "How have you been?"- No one wants to be used. Also, don't beat yourself up if some connections are lost. It is a part of growth. There are levels of connections and networking which I will discuss in more detail in a future writing. Using this plan helps create a relationship of mutual respect. Time is needed to build connections.

47

4. What should I know about night shift?

While I have not worked night shift, one of my friends did during her first year of nursing and told me night shift is different in that nurse autonomy is more so prevalent as provider rounds and patient care activities happen during the day. In fact, she found herself able to read during her down time on the shift after patient care needs were attended to.
Now this may not be the experience for everyone but it's a good point of reference.

I suggest interviewing and/or shadowing night shift nurses in different phases such as those just starting out, mid-way through the experience (3-5years), and veterans (5years and beyond) so you can ask lots of questions. Also, think about your sleeping schedule. How much and when do you like to sleep? Or you can look at it this way: What time of day are you most productive/ at your best? That's probably when you want to work if possible.

5. Will holding a PCT (Patient Care Tech) job prior to graduation increase my chances of RN position at graduation?

One of my nursing friends asked and answered a similar question to the above as follow: *"In my experience, it is not absolutely necessary but it is very helpful. Once you are hired as a PCT, your boss already knows you and [will] hire you if they have an opening rather than hiring a RN from [the] outside."*

I agree with the above answer and would add it depends on the place and/or hospital you are trying to work at after graduation. For example, my first job after graduation as you know was at a local health department. In this instance, working as a home health aide would not have afforded me the flexibility to go to school. I was still able to obtain the RN position I wanted without prior Patient Care Tech experience.

It is never too early to start planning your nursing career. For instance, I always planned to work in the public health field. It was more beneficial for me to focus on participating in public health activities such as flu drives and outreach while maintaining a more flexible schedule rather than working as a PCT before graduation. On the other hand, there is a very exclusive hospital in our area that usually only hires from within, I know several nurses that started out there as PCT 's and were easily/readily transitioned in as staff RNs. A little research can go a long way. See Lesson # 7.

6. What is the best way to obtain a job? *Through agencies? Online applications/social media, networking? In-person? Connections?*

It appears, from my experience the nursing field is and remaining more about who you know rather than what you know (Lesson #2). For that simple reason alone, please pay attention to who you are networking with. As we discussed earlier, this could make your career or place you several steps back. As you know networking and making connections is how I was introduced to my first public health nursing job.

I have also had success finding positions on the internet; a simple internet search can really do wonders. For example, if you want to be an ER or psychiatric nurse simply type in the search engine the desired position, title, and the desired location of employment, i.e. Psychiatric or mental health nurse Baltimore, MD. You will be amazed the amount of information you find from public, private, and governmental companies. Then, you just have to narrow it down. Personally, I had success with *www.simplyhired.com* and *www.indeed.com* these job search engines provide other key words related to desired position and allows you to create job alerts based on saved search parameters. There really is no one approach fits all. Sometimes a combination of the above or one of these methods will work, trust your gut and keep track of the method(s) that works for you and make that/ those methods as your point of reference when starting your job search.

7. What if I become overwhelmed by nursing school and need to take a break?

As you have or will learn in your required Public/Community Health nursing class, there are three levels of intervention; primary, secondary, and tertiary(Clark,2008). In this case, you can utilize these levels for your success.

Primary Level: Self-Care is important to prevent and protect yourself from becoming burnt out. You can only study and rewrite your patient care plans so much.

Secondary Level: If you are in the midst of a crisis seek counsel. Sometimes you need an outside trusted individual, support network, or professional that can help you regain perspective.

Tertiary Level: Once the initial crisis is over its time to maintain your inner peace and get back on track with preventive measures such as taking some time for fresh air and putting your crisis prevention plan in place

Burnout will happen at some point in your career and possibly more than once if you're not careful. I have been burnt out, down, depressed, sad, anxious, and unable to sleep due to being overwhelmed by the vastness and complexities of nursing. But I have learned how to maintain, navigate, and prevent the aftermath of emotions using the strategies in this book. Above all else, never underestimate the power of prayer!

The Bottom Line: We are all a work in progress, ask questions.

Bonus: My Crisis Prevention Plan©:

Kimberly Raquel Ward September 2011

Email: *raquiwardrn@gmail.com,* **Twitter:** *@RaquiWard*

LinkedIn: *Kimberly R. Ward*

The crisis prevention plan is something I personally use and hope you will too. In 2011 I came up with a plan for myself to more effectively deal with crisis, in my case due to work related stress. I subsequently presented this concept/ document during an educational group at my former employer and have since expanded to include the latter. The plan is broken up into three parts. First is the self-reflection section, this will help you analyze where you have been to know where you are going. I suggest doing this if at all possible before a crisis begins but I wrote this when I was in a crisis so I understand if that's when you do it too. Second, are the actual steps of your plan. I provided steps that I feel are all important as a part of a soundly founded Crisis Prevention Plan. The third section is how to practically implement your plan. I encourage you to write your plan down and keep it handy ☺

Self-Reflection:

1. When I have a crisis I:

2. Reactions to my crisis:

3. When I have a crisis I will:

4. Causes of my crisis:

<u>Steps</u>:

1. Recognize the signs of impeding crisis (what are the clues that something is about to happen?)

2. Take Care of myself regardless of how I'm feeling: i.e.: shower, rest, exercise

3. At work be cognizant of my surroundings and focus on the task at hand, one task at a time

4. Daily devotional- whether talking, reading, or writing about the Word.

5. Do physical activity or something with my hands that is not work related

6. Remind myself "I am only one person, I give my all but the rest is in God's hands."

7. Share my plan such as warning signs listed in self-reflection with someone I trust to keep me accountable/ look out for me in crisis.

Action/ Implementation of Plan: How can I practically integrate this plan into my life?

1. Review crisis prevention plan periodically, making updates/changes as needed based on new information gathered from previous crisis experiences

2. Share information with accountability partner, once crisis recognized, alert this person via code word or statement

3. Focus on one action you can tackle such as increase fluids progressing to other needs as necessary until then have accountability partner care for other needs.

4. Increase positivity in self-talk and surroundings

5. Remain fluid in crisis - except crisis for what it is, deal with the emotions attached to it, and then move on once you have worked it through.

6. Practice, Practice, Practice.

7. Once crisis completed move on to self-preservation mode, thank those who helped your through the crisis

8. Plan ahead as much as possible:

The goal is not to be perfect but recognize what works for you. There is no right way to deal in crisis. This is a guide to help you. Not all the information is needed for all crises some crises last longer than others or have a greater impact. Preparation is key. Eventually you'll be able to do this automatically when crisis happens.

Feel free to contact me for more ideas, tips, and/or with questions.

Scriptures to Inspire

Jeremiah 29:11

Hebrews 11:1-3

Philippians 4:16

Psalm 23

Galatians 6:9

Matthew 6:25-34

34:"Therefore do not worry about tomorrow, for tomorrow will worry about its own things. Sufficient for the day is its own trouble."

References:

1. Johnson & Johnson (2013). The Campaign For Nursing's Future. Explore Specialties. Retrieved September 19,2013, from http://www.discovernursing.com/explore-specialties#no-filters

2. Merriam-Webster Incorporated (2013). Retrieved September 23, 2013, from http://www.merriam-webster.com/

3. Ward, Raqui (2013, May 9). A Nurses Legacy [Web blog posting] Retrieved from http://horizions.blogspot.com/2013/05/a-nurses-legacy.html

4. Ward. Raqui (2010). New Beginnings [Web blog postings]. Horizions.blogspot.com

5. Ventus-Drakes, K. (2012, May).Women! Heal Thyself: Mind. Body, Spirit. In The Florida Minority Health Promotion Network Inc. (Host), *The Dr. Kim Experience.* Conference conducted from University Of South Florida, Tampa, FL.

6. Clark, M.J.D. (2008).Community Health Nursing: Advocacy for Population Health (5th Ed.). Upper Saddle River, New Jersey: Pearson Education, Inc.

7. Ward, K.R. (2011). *My Crisis Prevention Plan.* In Press.

8. Tyndale *Life Application Study Bible NKJV (*1996).Holy Bible NKJV (1982) by Thomas Nelson. Tyndale House Publishers Inc., Carol Stream, IL.

About:

Hi, I'm Kimberly, you may know me as Raqui(pronounced rocky) from my blog at horizions.blogspot.com or @Raquiward on Twitter where my goal is to encourage nurses 0-5 years into their career daily. I feel we as people spend too much time on the negative. I'm all about the positive. The only thing holding you back is **You**! I am a wife, mother, sister, daughter, Christ follower, public health nurse, and author. I am enjoying the journey of self-discovery and look forward to connecting with you.

As I said earlier I want to hear about you. Who you are, where you're from, how did you get into nursing, and what's your story, we all have a story. It's a matter of if, when, and who we choose to tell. You can connect with me on
Twitter:@RaquiWard
LinkedIn: Kimberly R. Ward or
Email: raquiwardrn@gmail.com

Take Care,

~ Kimberly